OVERCOMING DRUG ADDICTION

Simple and easy remedies to deal with drug addiction.

Laurence Payne

INTRODUCTION

Humans have been misusing drugs like meth, cocaine, nicotine, and marijuana for a very long time. Societies in China, the Middle East, and early America have documented consuming marijuana as far back as 5,000 BC. Cannabis sativa is a plant that grows wild all over the world and is used to make marijuana, which is a dried, shredded mixture of its flowers, stems, and leaves. As US state governments continue to progress the process of gradual legalization for medicinal prescription, marijuana has received a lot of media attention recently. Public cultivation and even consumption for leisure. Putting an end to the more than 40 years of federal legislation that prohibits it as a schedule.

even though the cannabis plant flowering stalk has shown to host a variety of medicinal properties that continue to be of benefit to people with a wide range of illnesses, including glaucoma, cancer, eating disorders, autism, and aches and pains from other diseases. It continues to hold the status of a schedule 1 controlled substance at the federal level in the United States.

Despite not having the dramatic physical signs of intoxication as alcohol and hard opioids do, wacky cannabis can nevertheless be overused, misused, and become addictive. Drug dependence that results in depression, anxiety, lack of motivation, and disassociation in the user has been demonstrated to develop with prolonged and frequent drug use.

According to a 1993 poll, substance misuse is a global epidemic in the United States alone.

Misuse of certain drugs, such as marijuana, meth, cocaine, or nicotine, is an example of drug addiction. Has been used by humans for a long time; societies in China, the Middle East, and early America have recorded smoking it as far back as 5,000 B.Ch.E. dried, the shredded mixture of flowers, stems, and leaves from the Cannabis Sativa plant, which can be found growing in the wild all over the world, is what we call marijuana. In recent times, the media in the United States has paid a lot of attention to marijuana as state governments continue to move forward with the gradual legalization of marijuana for medical use. Public cultivation and even consumption for pleasure. Effectively putting an end to federal legislation that has banned it as a schedule for more than 40 years.

Even though the cannabis plant is still classified as a Schedule 1 controlled substance at the federal level in the United States, the flowering stalk has been shown to contain several medicinal properties that continue to be beneficial to people who suffer from a wide range of ailments, such as glaucoma, cancer, eating disorders, autism, and the aches and pains caused by other diseases.

Even though wild marijuana does not exhibit the severe physical symptoms of intoxication that are associated with hard drugs and alcohol, it is still susceptible to abuse, misuse, and addiction. An addiction that leads to depression, anxiety, lack of motivation, and disassociation has been demonstrated to develop in users who use drugs regularly for an extended period.

In the United States alone, substance abuse is a global epidemic; a 1993 survey found that 14.5 million households were using illegal drugs and 40 million were heavy drinkers. In the past few decades, global tobacco use has increased by almost 75%.

In the United States, substance abuse is now the most common health issue and the leading cause of death. Alcohol is linked to more than 100,000 deaths annually. Cigarette smoking is the cause of one in six deaths.400, 000 people die annually as a result of smoking cigarettes, and another 50,000 die annually as a result of secondary smoke. One-third of all hospital admissions, 25% of all deaths, and the majority of serious crimes are thought to be linked to drug, alcohol, or cigarette addiction. Additionally, alcohol is linked to 25% of emergency room admissions and one-third of all suicides.

These figures only reflect the long-term effects and high costs of substance abuse. Millions more people worldwide suffer from behavioral or activity addictions that cause serious physical, psychological, occupational, financial, interpersonal, and compulsive behaviors like eating, gambling, sexual activity, working out, spending money, and using the internet. The word "compulsive" is emphasized. The drug war has not stopped the growing problem of substance abuse.

Although substance abuse has decreased in some instances both inside and outside of prisons, the majority of inmates do not receive treatment for substance abuse issues, with only 30% of inmates participating in rehabilitation programs.

Anxiety and depression are the other two mental health epidemics that are currently sweeping the world alongside addiction. The world is filled with depression and anxiety. In the second half of the 20th century, the prevalence of anxiety disorders skyrocketed to the point where they are now the most common "mental" illness.

One in nine Americans now has an anxiety disorder at any given time. The number of people suffering from depression is also rising at an alarming rate. In the United States alone, 30 million people are taking Prozac, which is now one of the top ten most commonly prescribed medications. This amounts to nearly one in ten people. A study conducted by the World Health Organization indicates that depression will be the single most common cause of death worldwide by the year 2000.

There has not been a parallel worldwide rise in addiction, anxiety, or depression. These are disorders that are intertwined rather than distinct epidemics. This book reveals that anxiety and depression are untreated disorders that explain the appalling statistics of traditional addiction treatment: therefore, 90% of drug and alcohol addicts and alcoholics relapse (the percentage varies depending on the statistical source); additionally, suicide accounts for almost 25% of the deaths of chemical dependency treatment patients.

A review of comparative studies of standard treatment approaches, including Alcoholics Anonymous, revealed that there is little or no evidence of effectiveness. Although twelve-step programs like Alcoholics Anonymous and others make a valuable contribution by providing peer support and a structure for addiction recovery,

, depression and anxiety have both been linked to suicide.

Marijuana, for instance, is hardly comparable to the more destructive drugs on the market, such as cocaine, meth, and heroin. The effects of cannabis are subtle and include a calm euphoria, increased empathy, and a tendency to encourage relaxed and associative thought patterns. Cannabis users, on the other hand, find themselves stuck in this situation and have little desire to escape.

It is essential to differentiate between a frequent smoker who prefers not to go more than a few hours without a fix and someone who has only tried cannabis a few times.

If you don't already believe in destiny, I strongly encourage you to reconsider your life there are certain discernible chains of events that cannot be discounted as mere coincidence for the sake of arguments there are two distinct forms of destiny, which you make happen and that which happens to you. If you don't already believe in destiny, I strongly urge you to reconsider your life there are certain discernible chains of events that cannot be discounted as mere coincidence for the sake of argument sit is simple to conclude in hindsight that your particular set of circumstances predestined you to become a drug addict. It took place. You must now decide whether or not you are destined to become an ex-drug addict. This is the kind of destiny you can create, but true destiny is a combination of what happens to you and what you create.

As a band member, I was an addict at the time. Meth had affected us and made it impossible for us to naturally function as a unit; not long after that, meth made it impossible for me to function as an individual. Everyone predicted that I would lose everything, and I did. My dignity, my pride, my house, my family, and my car.

We all went through the same things at this point. Don't you believe it when people say that different people react differently? We all acted the same way when we used meth, and our genetic personality trait sometimes makes it appear different, but we are all the same. We are bound to face the same struggle.

Addiction to drugs is categorically a death wish. The daily torture of self-medication is accompanied by a sober determination to stop using sooner rather than later when casual use develops into chemical dependency. You will eventually realize that quitting completely is the only thing that can save your life. As a result, you consider the major query: Do I need to leave for something? If you don't have a clear motivation, your attempt to quit will only ever be an attempt. To define your motivation, you need to know what you want to quit.

Addiction to drugs is the easiest thing for anyone to do. It doesn't take much effort at all and gives you all the good reasons to be a failure.

This is just the beginning of a lengthy book that will take you through every aspect of your addiction journey. It will help you comprehend one of the factors that led to your addiction to drugs and, in the end, teach you how to overcome this obstacle.

Addiction to drugs is the primary distinction between drug use and chemical dependence. Addiction develops over time when the body's own capacity to develop a tolerance level reduces the drug's initial effects and necessitates a large dose to achieve the desired high. Your body adapts to the chemical as if it were designed to work with it in your system as you increase the number of drugs you take in, putting toxic levels of drugs into your bloodstream and eventually altering its chemistry.

The issue is that your body can no longer function without the chemical when you try to remove it.

To function normally or maintain a normal state, it now depends on that chemical. You are addicted because of this chemical dependence. If you try to stop taking the drug while you are chemically dependent, the cycle is obvious. There will be withdrawal symptoms for you. Your body is currently attempting to function without the medication. Your central nervous system is shocked in the same way it was when you first gave your body the drug. When you feel normal, everything you think and feel is completely different. That is the meaning of withdrawal. You are removing a chemical from your body that it currently requires to function normally. Since withdrawal is the most serious aspect of addiction, likely, you've already experienced them. Quitting is a terrible experience that has a simple cure: This pain will subside if you take your medication.

There are only three real strategies for breaking free of drug addiction. One is to quit on your own, the other is to go to a costly drug treatment center where all they do is lock you in a room, just like in a jail, and the third is to go to jail, where you can't get large doses of the drug. The third option, quitting on your own, is the most common and also the most difficult because you know where to easily obtain some of your drugs. Quitting is easy in a locked treatment facility or jail because you have no choice. When you leave in an altered state of consciousness, your sub consciousness may sometimes

A person, you're' a purchaser. Your body works related to your mind to accomplish its essential objective of being content. Thusly the body's activities should fulfill the cerebrum. As you probably are aware, we eat food and drink fluids to supply our body with essential enhancements to keep a solid way of life so we can live a long life. In this cycle, our mind and body fill in collectively and will generally believe each other's senses and we start the most common way of closing down and getting the important rest expects to work for the following waking time frame when the body is deficient with regards to an essential enhancement, the cerebrum sorts out what's required and utilizes the body to secure that component. For example, on the off chance that your body was deficient with regards to a legitimate inventory of L-ascorbic acid, the cerebrum could send the body to the store to get an orange, or possibly that is how it should work.

Sadly with the presentation of a compound into our bodies in pill structure, we have not just sorted out some way to ease our diseases quicker and all the more proficiently however we've likewise developed a more elevated level of trust between our bodies and our brain.

Illicit drug use isn't a sickness. Simply ask anybody who has at any point attempted to kick malignant growth. As a junkie, you have choices that just aren't accessible to somebody experiencing a difficult disease. You can stop. You can continue to accept you're a captive to chronic drug use, that there is no expectation, you'll constantly be a disappointment or you can stop, individuals who accept that illicit drug use is a sickness are pushed beyond their limits attempting to comprehend the reason why they or someone they know is as yet experiencing a chronic drug use when all method for understanding and therapy have been depleted.

This book offers a scope of treatment ways to deal with addressing these elements and genuinely reestablish wellbeing. Simply by considering the prosperity of the body, brain and soul could complete mending assume at any point position, which is confirmed by the far higher achievement pace of this model.

The book covers various sorts of approaches to defeating illicit drug use and a portion of these kinds of compulsion is committed to investigating the fundamental causal and contributing elements, fully intent on mending from fixation, as opposed to tolerating the lifetime mark of alcoholic or junkie. To this end, the book offers a scope of treatment ways to deal with addressing these variables and reestablishing wellbeing. Exclusively considering the prosperity of the body, psyche and soul could exhaustive recuperating assumes at any point position.

Every one of the treatments covered here approaches the treatment of dependence along these lines. They all offer the qualities of fitting treatment to the person, which is one more component for a fruitful result.

Section one starts with chronic drug use, the way things are being mishandled, and resilience. It additionally discusses justifications for why individuals with substance use jumble need increasingly more medication over the long run. Who is in danger of substance use jumble? How should substance utilize jumble influence me?

Section two examines about side effects and reasons for illicit drug use, why individuals consume medications, side effects of chronic drug use, finding and test, the executives and therapy, counteraction, and visualization.

Section three discusses living with chronic drug use and how best individuals living with illicit drug use can figure out how to deal with themselves.

Part four discusses conquering chronic drug use, solid ways of adapting to pressure, how to adapt to tranquilize desires, and holding your medication desires within proper limits.

Section five discusses ask surf; many individuals attempt to adapt to their desires by enduring it and essential steps of urge surfing and building a significant medication-free life.

Part six discusses amino corrosive treatment, what are amino acids, how amino corrosive habit treatment work, and how might I benefit from amino corrosive treatment.

Section seven examines the actual sensitivities of dependence and liquor and aversion to any substance, drug sensitivities, for what reason truly do sedate sensitivities occur, and what medication causes the most medication sensitivities.

Section eight discusses homegrown solutions for illicit drug use and the ways to deal with a social treatment that the junkie can attempt.

CHAPTER ONE

What is illicit drug use?

Dependence is a sickness that influences your cerebrum and conduct. At the point when you're dependent on drugs, you can't fight the temptation to utilize them, regardless of how much mischief the medications might cause. The prior you seek treatment for illicit drug use, the almost certain you are to stay away from a portion of the more desperate outcomes of the infection.

Chronic drug use isn't about heroin, cocaine, or other unlawful medications. You can get dependent on liquor, nicotine, rest, and hostile to tension meds, and other lawful substances.

You can likewise get dependent on remedy or unlawfully acquired opiate torment meds, or narcotics. This problem is at epidemic positions in the US. In 2018, narcotics assumed a part in 66% of all medication glut passing.

From the beginning, you might decide to take medication since you like how it causes you to feel. You might figure you have some control over how much and how frequently you use it. In any case, over the long run, drugs change how your cerebrum works. These actual changes can keep going for quite a while. They cause you to let completely go and can prompt harmful ways of behaving.

Habit versus Misuse and Resistance

Chronic drug use is the point at which you utilize lawful or unlawful substances in manners you shouldn't. You could take more than the standard portion of pills or use another person's remedy. You might manhandle medications to feel better, ease pressure, or keep away from the real world. Be that as it may, typically, you're ready to address your unfortunate things to do or quit utilizing out and out.

Habit is the point at which you can't stop. Not when it jeopardizes your well-being. Not when it causes monetary, close to home, and different issues for you or your friends and family. That inclination to get and utilize medications can top off each moment of the day, regardless of whether you need to stop.

Enslavement likewise is not the same as actual reliance or resistance. In instances of actual reliance, withdrawal side effects happen when you out of nowhere stop a substance. Resilience happens when a portion of a substance turns out to be less viable over the long haul.

At the point when you use narcotics for torment for quite a while, for instance, you might foster resilience and, surprisingly, actual reliance. This doesn't mean you're dependent. As a rule, when opiates are utilized under legitimate clinical management, fixation occurs in just a little level of individuals

What medications lead to habit?

Drugs that are ordinarily abused include:

Liquor.

Club drugs, similar to GHB, ketamine, MDMA (happiness/molly), and flunitrazepam (Rohypnol®).

Energizers, like cocaine (counting break) and methamphetamine (meth).

Stimulants, including ayahuasca, D-lysergic corrosive diethylamide (LSD), peyote (mescaline), phencyclidine (PCP), and DMT.

Inhalants, including solvents, spray showers, gases, and nitrites (poppers).

Maryjane.

Narcotic pain relievers like heroin, fentanyl, oxycodone, hydrocodone, codeine, and morphine.

Doctor-prescribed medications and cold prescriptions.

Narcotics, hypnotics, and anxiolytics (against nervousness prescriptions).

Steroids (anabolic).

Engineered cannabinoids (K2 or Flavor).

Manufactured cotinine (shower salts).

Tobacco/nicotine and electronic cigarettes (e-cigarettes or vaping).

While these medications are different from one another, they all unequivocally enact the habit focus of the mind. That is the very thing that makes these substances propensity shaping, while others are not.

For what reason in all actuality do individuals with substance utilize jumble need an ever-increasing number of medications over the long run?

Individuals feel inebriated after utilizing drugs. After some time, the mind is changed by drugs. The mind becomes desensitized to the medication so a greater amount of the medication should be utilized to deliver a similar outcome.

As the individual consumes more, drugs begin to assume control over the individual's life. One might quit appreciating different parts of life. For some reason, there are some, social, family, and work commitments that collapse. The individual with SUD begins to feel like something's off-base on the off chance that the person in question isn't affected by the substance. They might become consumed with the need to recover that unique inclination.

CHAPTER TWO

Who is in danger of substance use jumble?

Anybody can foster a substance use jumble. Nobody thing can foresee whether an individual might foster a habit. You might be more inclined to medicate use due to:

Science: The individual's hereditary cosmetics, orientation, nationality, and emotional wellness issues might raise their gamble of fostering a compulsion. Around 66% of individuals in habit treatment are men. Specific nationalities are at higher gamble for substance use jumble. This is valid for Local Americans.

Climate: Environmental factors can influence the probability of creating a substance use jumble. For instance, stress, peer pressure, physical or sexual maltreatment, and early openness to medications can raise the gamble.

Age: Teens who begin ingesting medications are particularly in danger. The pieces of the cerebrum that control judgment, choices, and restraint are not completely evolved. Youngsters are bound to participate in hazardous ways of behaving. In a creating cerebrum, medications can cause changes that make the habit more probable.

How normal is drug used jumble?

Drug substance and liquor are the main sources used to prevent sickness and early demise. Research has shown that around 1 out of 9 Americans utilize sporting medications (around 11% of the populace). The most regularly abused drugs are weed and physician-recommended meds.

How should substance utilize jumble influence me?

Drugs influence the cerebrum, particular

How might I be affected by substance abuse disorder?

The "reward center" of the brain is especially affected by drugs.

The biological drive to seek rewards drives humans. These rewards frequently result from healthy actions. Your body makes a chemical called dopamine, which makes you feel good when you spend time with a loved one or eat something delicious. It turns into a loop: Because these experiences give you good feelings, you seek them out.

Dopamine is also transported massively throughout the brain by drugs. However, such high levels of dopamine can cause detrimental changes in thoughts, feelings, and behavior rather than motivating you to do the things you need to do to survive—eat, work, and spend time with loved ones—because you won't feel motivated to do them. That can lead to an unhealthy desire to seek drug-induced pleasure and less for more healthy pleasures. The cycle centers on seeking out and using drugs to experience a pleasure.

Over time, drug addiction alters the brain. It has an impact on the brain's structure as well as its workings. Because of this, medical professionals consider substance abuse disorders to be brain diseases.

A drug's first use is a choice. However, addiction has the potential to develop into a very dangerous condition. Your ability to make decisions, including the decision to stop using drugs, is affected by drugs.

You might be aware of the issue but unable to stop. Stopping drug use can be physically uncomfortable for addicts. It has the potential to harm you and even put your life in danger.

SYMPTOMS AND CAUSES The purpose of drug use

People use drugs for many obvious reasons they might:

Take pleasure in the experience.

Desire to alleviate or alter their negative emotions.

Want to perform better at work, in school, or in sports.

Choose to resist peer pressure or be curious.

What signs and symptoms does a substance use disorder have?

The following are signs of drug addiction:

Eyes that are bloodshot and tired.

Changes in appetite, typically with less eating.

Changes in how you look, like having a bad complexion or not grooming yourself.

A need for drugs.

Difficulty finishing tasks at home, at work, or in school.

Even though they are aware of the potential negative consequences, such as driving while impaired or having sex without protection

Powerlessness to diminish or control drug use.

Problems with money

Shedding pounds.

How are substance use disorders diagnosed and tested?

Recognizing the issue and wanting assistance is the first step in obtaining a drug addiction diagnosis. An intervention from friends or loved ones might be the first step in this process following the reasons why individuals need to make a decision to go for treatment

Complete a healthcare provider's examination.

Personalized care, whether in or out-patient.

MANAGEMENT AND TREATMENT

What are drug addiction treatments?

There are several treatments for substance use disorders. Treatment can be beneficial even in severe cases. You might get a combination of these treatments:

Detoxification: You stop using drugs and let the drugs out of your body. To detox safely, medical supervision may be required.

Therapies supported by medication: Medicine can help control cravings and alleviate withdrawal symptoms during detox.

Behavior therapies: The root cause of addiction can be addressed with cognitive behavioral therapy or other psychotherapy (talk therapy). Therapy also teaches healthy coping strategies and boosts self-esteem.

What medications can be used to treat substance abuse?

Your treatment plan may include medication. The best medications for you are determined by your care team. Treatments with medication assistance are available for:

Opioids: For the treatment of opiate use disorder, the FDA has approved methadone, buprenorphine, and naltrexone.

Alcohol: Naltrexone, acamprosate, and disulfiram (Antabuse®) are three drugs that have been approved by the FDA.

Tobacco: A nicotine lozenge, spray, patch, or spray can be helpful. Additionally, bupropion (Wellbutrin®) or varenicline (Chantix®) may be prescribed by your physician.

Is there outpatient or inpatient drug addiction treatment?

Depending on your requirements, treatment options include both inpatient and outpatient settings. From three months to a year, treatment typically consists of weekly group therapy sessions.

Some examples of inpatient therapy are:

Hospitalization.

Sober houses or therapeutic communities are tightly controlled drug-free settings.

As you undergo treatment, there are some groups such as Alcoholics Anonymous and Narcotics Anonymous that can be of help. Al-Anon and Nar-Anon Family Groups are two examples of family-oriented self-help groups. It has been demonstrated that participating in 12-step-based recovery work improves outcomes.

Is substance abuse disorder treatable?

Drug addiction does not have a treatment. Addiction can be managed and treated. However, there is always the possibility of the addiction resurfacing. It takes a lifetime to manage a substance use disorder.

PREVENTION is it possible to prevent substance abuse disorders?

Yes. Education is the first step in preventing drug addiction. Community, family, and school education all play a role in preventing first-time substance abuse. Other strategies for avoiding substance abuse disorders:

Even if you try illegal drugs once, never again.

When taking prescription drugs, follow the directions. Never take more than what is directed. For instance, opioid addiction can begin within five days.

Reduce the likelihood that others will misuse unused prescriptions by disposing of them promptly.

Are there conditions that increase the likelihood of developing a substance use disorder?

A lot of people suffer from both mental health issues and substance use disorders. Occasionally, mental illness exists before addiction. Sometimes, the addiction causes or makes a mental health problem worse. The likelihood of recovery increases when both conditions are treated appropriately.

PROGNOSIS / OUTLOOK how do people with substance use disorders fare in the future?

The disease of addiction lasts a lifetime. However, addiction can be overcome and people can live full lives. Recovery requires getting help. Some people benefit from various tools, but others benefit from ongoing therapy and self-help groups like Narcotics Anonymous.

CHAPTER THREE

Does addiction have lasting effects?

The structures and functions of the brain can change if you continue to use drugs. Having a substance use disorder affects how you:

Behave.

Manage stress.

Learn.

Make decisions and judgments.

Maintain memories.

Is addiction reversible?

A "relapsing disease" is a substance use disorder. People who have recovered from this illness are more likely to use drugs again. Even years after you last took drugs, recurrence can occur.

How might substance abuse disorder affect me?

Drugs have a particular effect on the brain's "reward center."

Humans are driven by the biological need to seek out rewards. Healthy actions frequently lead to these rewards. When you eat something delectable or spend time with a loved one, your body produces a chemical called dopamine, which makes you feel good. It becomes a loop: You look for these positive experiences because they make you feel good.

Drugs also significantly transport dopamine throughout the brain. However, having such high levels of dopamine can have the opposite effect of motivating you to do the things you need to do to survive—eat, work, and spend time with loved ones—because you won't feel motivated to do them. Instead, it can cause negative changes in thoughts, feelings, and behavior. That may result in an unhealthy desire to seek drug-induced pleasure rather than healthier pleasures. The focus of the cycle is on seeking pleasure through drug use.

Addiction to drugs alters the brain over time. It affects how the brain works and how it is built.

Medical professionals, therefore, classify substance abuse disorders as brain diseases.

The decision to use drugs in the first place is a choice. Addiction, on the other hand, has the potential to become a very dangerous condition. Drugs affect your decision-making abilities, including your ability to stop using drugs.

You might be aware of the problem, but you can't stop yourself. Addicts may experience physical discomfort when they stop using drugs. It could hurt you or even put your life in danger.

SYMPTOMS AND CAUSES The goal of drug use there are numerous motivations for drug use. They may:

Enjoy the experience to the fullest.

Desire to change or lessen their negative feelings.

Desire to improve their performance at work, in school, or in sports.

Choose to be curious or resist peer pressure.

What are substance use disorders' signs and symptoms?

Addiction to drugs can be seen in the following ways:

Tired eyes with a bloodshot appearance.

Changes in appetite, typically accompanied by fewer meals.

Changes in your appearance, such as a poor complexion or a lack of self-care.

A desire to use drugs

Difficulties completing assignments at home, at work, and in school.

Even though they are aware of the potential negative outcomes, such as driving while impaired or engaging in sexual activity without protection, they cannot reduce or control their drug use.

Problems with money disappearing.

What methods are used to test for and diagnose substance use disorders?

The first step in getting a drug addiction diagnosis is recognizing the problem and wanting help. The first step in this process might be an intervention from friends or family. The following are the consequences of an individual's decision to seek addiction treatment:

Obtain an examination from a healthcare professional.

Individualized care, whether in or out of the hospital.

How are drug addiction treatments managed and treated?

Substance abuse disorders can be treated in several different ways. Even in severe cases, treatment can be beneficial. You might get all of these treatments at once:

Detoxification: You get rid of the drugs and stop using them. Medical supervision may be required for safe detox.

Medication-supported treatments: During detox, medication can help control cravings and ease withdrawal symptoms.

Behavior therapies: Cognitive behavioral therapy or other psychotherapy (talk therapy) can address the underlying cause of addiction. It also teaches healthy coping mechanisms and boosts self-esteem.

What drugs are available to treat substance abuse?

Medication may be included in your treatment plan. Your care team will decide which medications are best for you. For the following conditions, medication assistance is available:

Opioids: The FDA has approved methadone, buprenorphine, and naltrexone for opiate use disorder treatment.

Alcohol: The FDA has approved naltrexone, acamprosate, and disulfiram (Antabuse®) as medications.

Tobacco: A nicotine spray, lozenge, or spray can be beneficial. Your doctor may also prescribe bupropion (Wellbutrin®) or varenicline (Chantix®).

Is there a choice between outpatient and inpatient drug addiction treatment?

Treatment options include both inpatient and outpatient settings, depending on your needs. Treatment typically consists of weekly group therapy sessions for three months to a year.

Inpatient therapy can look like the following:

Hospitalization.

Drug-free settings like sober houses or therapeutic communities are tightly controlled.

Self-help groups like Alcoholics Anonymous and Narcotics Anonymous can be helpful on the road to recovery. Family-focused self-help groups include Al-Anon and Nar-Anon Family Groups. Participation in 12-step-based recovery programs has been shown to improve outcomes.

Can addiction to substances be treated?

There is no cure for drug addiction. There are ways to control and treat addiction. However, relapse into addiction is always a possibility. Managing a substance use disorder takes a lifetime.

PREVENTION Can substance abuse disorders be avoided?

Yes. Preventing drug addiction begins with education. Education in the community, the family, and the school all contribute to the prevention of first-time substance abuse. Other ways to stay away from substance abuse disorders:

Never try illegal drugs again, even once.

Always adhere to the label when taking prescription medications. Never take more than your prescription. Opioid addiction, for instance, can begin within five days.

By disposing of them promptly, you can lower the likelihood that other people will misuse unused prescriptions.

Are there circumstances that are associated with an increased risk of developing a substance abuse disorder?

Numerous individuals struggle with both substance use disorders and mental health issues. Sometimes, mental illness comes before addiction. Addiction can sometimes lead to or exacerbate mental health issues. When both conditions are treated appropriately, recovery is more likely.

PROGNOSIS / OUTLOOK how do substance abusers fare in the future?

Addiction is a disease that lasts a lifetime. Addiction, on the other hand, can be overcome, and people can live full lives. Recovery necessitates assistance. Various tools help some people, while ongoing therapy and self-help groups like Narcotics Anonymous help others.

Is addiction a chronic condition?

If you continue to use drugs, the brain's structures and functions may change. A substance use disorder has an impact on how you:

Behave.

Reduce stress.

Learn.

Make judgments and decisions.

Keep your memories.

Can addiction be reversed?

Substance use disorder is a "relapsing disease. It is more likely that people who have recovered from this illness will use drugs again. Recurrence can occur even years after you last took drugs.

CHAPTER FOUR

Overcoming Drug Addiction Are you prepared to address your substance abuse issue? You can overcome your substance use disorder, deal with cravings, and prevent relapse with this step-by-step guide.

The first step toward overcoming drug abuse and addiction Drug addiction is not a sign of weakness or a character flaw; rather, it requires more than willpower to overcome the issue. Abusing prescription or illegal drugs can alter the brain, leading to intense cravings and a compulsion to use that makes sobriety seem impossible. However, regardless of how hopeless your situation appears or how many times you have tried and failed, recovery is always within reach. Change is always attainable with the appropriate treatment and assistance.

The very first step on the path to recovery is often the most difficult for many people who are struggling with addiction: recognizing a problem and making the decision to change its normal to be unsure of your readiness to begin recovery or whether you have what it takes to quit. If you are addicted to a prescription drug, you might be worried about how you will treat a medical condition differently. It's alright to be split up. Many things must be altered to commit to sobriety, including:

How you deal with stress, who you let into your life, what you do in your spare time, how you feel about yourself, and the prescription and over-the-counter medications you take. It's also normal to be conflicted about giving up your preferred drug, even if you know it's causing problems for you. You can overcome your addiction and regain control of your life by committing to change, but recovery takes time, motivation, and support.

Change is in the air. Keep track of when and how much you use drugs. You will have a better understanding of how the addiction is affecting your life as a result of this.

Make a list of the advantages and disadvantages of continuing to use drugs, as well as the costs and benefits of quitting.

Take into consideration the things that are significant to you, such as your health, your career, your children, or your pets. What effects does taking drugs to have on those things?

Discuss your drug use with someone you can trust.

Consider whether there is anything that prevents you from making changes. What might assist you in making the change?

Getting ready for change: Five keys to recovery from addiction: Remind yourself of your motivations for making the change.

Consider any previous attempts at recovery you may have made. What did work? Which did not?

Set goals that are specific and measurable, like a start date or drug usage limits.

De-stuff your home, place of employment, and other places you frequent with no remembrance of your addiction.

Consider any previous attempts at recovery you may have made. What did work? Which did not?

Set goals that are specific and measurable, like a start date or drug usage limits.

De-stuff your home, place of employment, and other places you frequent with no remembrance of your addiction.

Make a commitment to recovery for your loved ones and ask for their support.

After you have committed to recovery, it is time to investigate your treatment options. A successful addiction treatment program frequently incorporates several different components, such as:

Detoxification. Usually, the first thing you need to do is get rid of drugs and deal with withdrawal symptoms.

Behavioral therapy. You can learn healthier coping strategies, repair your relationships, and identify the underlying causes of your drug use through an individual, group, or family therapy.

Any co-occurring mental health condition, such as depression or anxiety, can be treated with medication, withdrawal symptoms can be controlled, and relapse prevention can be achieved.

Maintaining sobriety and preventing relapse can both be aided by long-term follow-up. To assist you in maintaining your recovery on track, this may include regularly attending online or in-person support groups.

Types of drug treatment program Residential treatment: While receiving intensive treatment, residential treatment entails living in a facility away from work, school, family, and other addiction triggers. Treatment in a residential setting can last anywhere from a few days to months.

Day treatment or partial hospitalization: People who want to continue living at home while maintaining a stable living environment are eligible for partial hospitalization. Typically, these programs meet at a treatment center for seven to eight hours each day, and you return home at night.

Outpatient treatment: These outpatient programs can be scheduled around work or school, and they are not residential. You are treated during the day or night, but you are not there overnight. Prevention of relapse is the primary focus.

Sober living communities: Typically, an intensive treatment program, such as residential treatment, is followed by living in a sober house. You live in a drug-free, safe environment with other recovering addicts. If you don't know where to go or are worried that going back home too soon will cause you to relapse, sober living facilities can help.

Tips for selecting the best drug addiction treatment keep in mind that no treatment is right for everyone. Everybody has different requirements. Addiction treatment should be tailored to your particular circumstances, regardless of whether you have a problem with a prescription or illegal drugs. Finding a program that feels right is critical.

More than just your drug abuse should be addressed in treatment. Your relationships, career, health, and psychological well-being are all affected by addiction. Changing your way of life and addressing the root causes of your drug use are essential to treatment success. You may need to find a healthier way to alleviate pain or cope with stressful situations if, for instance, your drug dependency stems from a desire to manage pain or stress.

The key is to commit and follow through. Treatment for drug addiction is not a simple or quick process. In general, the more time and effort you put into using drugs, the more treatment you'll need. In addition, long-term follow-up care is essential to recovery in all instances.

There are numerous resources available to you. A prolonged stay in rehab or medically supervised detox is not necessary for everyone. Your age, drug use history, and medical or psychiatric conditions all play a role in the care you require. Numerous clergy members, social workers, and counselors provide addiction treatment services in addition to doctors and psychologists.

Concurrently seek treatment for any mental health issues. In addition to seeking treatment for drug addiction, it is essential to address any other mental or physical issues you may be having. If you receive treatment for addiction and mental health from the same provider or team, you will have the best chance of recovery.

Recovery from addiction requires support; don't try to do it on your own. It is essential to have positive influences and a solid support system, regardless of the treatment method you choose. The more people you can turn to for support, direction, and a listening ear, the more likely it is that you will recover.

Rely on close family and friends. In the process of recovery, having the support of loved ones is an invaluable asset. Consider attending family therapy or relationship counseling if you are hesitant to turn to your loved ones because you have disappointed them in the past.

Establish a sober social circle. You may need to establish new connections if your previous social life was centered on drugs. Having sober friends who will help you recover is essential. Try attending events in your community, volunteering, taking a class, joining a church or civic group, or volunteering.

Think about moving into a home for sober people. During your recovery from drug addiction, sober living homes provide a secure and supportive environment. If you don't have a safe home or a drug-free environment, they're a good choice.

Prioritize meeting attendance. Attend meetings regularly and join a 12-step recovery support group like Narcotics Anonymous (NA). It can be very healing to spend time with people who know exactly what you're going through. You can also learn from the group members shared experiences and what they did to stay sober.

[Read: Assistance Groups: Types, Benefits, and What to Expect] Learn healthy ways to deal with stress after dealing with your addiction's immediate issues and beginning treatment, you'll still need to seek for solution concerning how the drug abuse all started. Did you start using it to calm down after an argument, relax after a bad day, forget about your problems, or numb painful emotions?

The negative emotions that you suppressed with drugs will return once you're clean. For treatment to be effective, you must first address your underlying issues.

You will occasionally continue to experience stress, loneliness, frustration, rage, shame, anxiety, and hopelessness even after your underlying issues have been resolved. All of these feelings are normal and part of life. A crucial part of your treatment and recovery is finding ways to deal with these emotions as they arise.

There are healthier methods for managing your stress. Without returning to your addiction, you can learn to manage your problems. When you are confident in your ability to de-stress quickly, confronting difficult emotions is less intimidating and overwhelming.

Drug-free methods for quickly reducing stress various methods for reducing stress work better for some people than for others. Finding the one that works best for you is the key.

Movement. Stress can be alleviated by taking a quick walk around the block. Additionally, yoga and meditation are excellent methods for reducing stress and achieving equilibrium.

Step outside and enjoy the fresh air and warm sun. Take in a breathtaking landscape or view.

Have fun with your cat or dog. Take pleasure in the soothing feel of your pet's fur.

Use your sense of smell to experiment. Breathe in the scent of freshly cut flowers or coffee beans, or enjoy the scent of sunscreen or a seashell that takes you back to a favorite vacation.

Imagine a tranquil setting with your eyes closed. Consider a cherished memory, such as your child's first steps or time spent with friends, or a sandy beach.

Treat yourself. Massage your neck or shoulders while you make yourself a steaming cup of tea. Take a warm shower or bath to soak.

Keep drug urges and triggers under control your recovery does not end when you become sober. Your brain still needs some time to recover and reestablish the connections that were altered while you were addicted. Drug cravings can be intense during this rebuilding process. Avoiding people, places, and circumstances that give you the urge to use can help you continue your recovery:

Get away from your drug-using friends. Stay away from friends who are still abusing drugs. You should surround yourself with people who are supportive of your sobriety rather than those who might tempt you to revert to old, harmful behaviors.

Avoid nightclubs and bars. Drinking lowers inhibitions and impairs judgment, which can easily lead to relapse even if you don't have a problem with alcohol. Drugs are frequently readily available, and the urge to use them can be strong. Also, stay away from any other places and situations that you think are associated with drug use.

When seeking medical care, be honest about any drug use you have had in the past. Be upfront and find a provider who will collaborate with you to either prescribe alternatives or the bare minimum of medication if you require a dental or medical procedure. You should never be denied pain medication or feel embarrassed or humiliated about using drugs in the past; if that occurs, look for a different provider.

Take prescription medications with caution. You may need to talk to your doctor about finding other ways to manage pain if you were addicted to a prescription drug, like an opioid painkiller. Regardless of the drug you had problems with, it's important to avoid prescription drugs that can be abused or only use them when necessary. Painkillers, sleeping pills, and anxiety medications are examples of drugs with a high risk of abuse.

How to deal with drug cravings Sometimes cravings can't be avoided, so you need to find a way to deal with them:

Challenge and alter your perspective. Many people, when they have a craving, tend to focus only on the benefits of the drug and forget about the drawbacks. As a result, it might be helpful to remind yourself that using won't make you feel better and that you stand to lose a lot. Keeping a small card with these consequences written down can sometimes be helpful.

CHAPTER FIVE

Immediately surf. By persevering, many people try to control their urges. But some cravings can't be ignored. Staying with the urge until it passes can be helpful in this situation. Urge surfing is the name of this strategy. Think of yourself as a surfer who will ride the wave of your drug craving, staying on top of it until it breaks into smaller, foamy waves. You'll notice that the craving passes more quickly than you think when you ride it out without fighting, judging, or ignoring it.

The three fundamental phases of urge surfing:

Pay attention to how you feel about the craving. Relax your hands and sit in a comfortable chair with your feet flat on the ground. Focus on your body as you take a few deep breaths. Take note of the location and sensations of the craving or urge in your body. Describe what you're feeling in words. You could, for instance, tell yourself: My craving is in my stomach, mouth, and nose.

Concentrate on a single area where you are craving something. What sensations do you experience there? Write them down for yourself. Take, for instance, the sensations of numbness, tingling, or heat. Perhaps your muscles are tight. How big of an area is it? As you focus on the sensations, observe if they change. My lips are dry. My lips are feeling numb. I can imagine the sensation of using it as I swallow.

Focusing on each area of your body that feels the urge, repeat. Give yourself a description of how the sensations change and how the urge comes and goes. After a few minutes of urge surfing, many people notice that their craving has gone away. However, the goal of this exercise is not to stop the urge, but rather to experience it in a new way

It will become easier for you to ride out your cravings until they naturally subside if you regularly engage in urge surfing.

Create a life without drugs that has meaning you can support your drug treatment and avoid relapse by engaging in activities and interests that give your life meaning. Being involved in activities that excite you, make you feel needed, and give your life meaning is crucial. Your addiction will lose its appeal when your life is filled with activities that give you satisfaction and a sense of purpose.

Take up an old pastime or try something new. Do activities that test your imagination and creativity—something you've always wanted to try. Try a new sport, learn a new language, or play a musical instrument.

Take in a pet. Although taking care of an animal makes you feel loved and needed, having a pet is a responsibility. Pets can also get you moving outside the house.

Spend time outdoors. Go camping, fishing, taking a scenic hike, or going for regular walks in a park.

Embrace the arts. Take a class in art, go to a concert or play, visit a museum, or write a memoir.

Engage in community service. Find drug-free groups and activities to replace your addiction. Participate as a volunteer, get involved in your faith community or church, or join a club or neighborhood group.

Set goals that matter. Antidotes to drug addiction include having objectives to work toward and something to look forward to. It doesn't matter what the objectives are; all that matters is that you value them.

Take care of your health. You can keep your energy levels up and your stress levels down by exercising regularly, getting enough sleep, and eating well. It will be easier for you to stay sober the more you can do to maintain your health and feel good.

CHAPTER SIX

Amino acid therapy the human body requires amino acids to carry out essential functions. Amino acids can be found all over the body. People who struggle with substance use disorders may also benefit from amino acids.

Amino acids come in many different varieties, each of which serves a distinct purpose. Some amino acids are essential, necessitating supplementation or food intake because the body cannot produce them on its own. The body can produce other amino acids on its own because they are non-essential.

Recovery from addiction relies heavily on amino acids. They aid in the body's reconstruction and regaining equilibrium. Additionally, they assist in reducing stress and anxiety, which are typical issues for individuals in recovery.

Because of this, Coalition Recovery offers our amino acid therapy program to clients who are having difficulty breaking free of alcohol or drug addiction. It is one of several treatments that are supported by evidence and provide relief to people who have been diagnosed with a substance use disorder.

AMINO ACIDS: WHAT ARE THEY?

Essential neurotransmitters, which are chemicals that contribute to addictive behavior, are built from amino acids. Various proteins that are essential to biology make up about 20% of the human body. These proteins are built on amino acids, which are also involved in numerous cellular processes and activities.

Alcohol and drugs typically alter brain chemistry by causing excessive production of neurotransmitters like dopamine. The subsequent rush of pleasure may signal the beginning of dependency issues that may develop into an addiction.

Your brain develops a drug dependence when you continue to abuse drugs. Because your amino acid balance is off, it forgets how to regulate different levels of neurotransmitters. When you take in a certain amount of alcohol or drugs, your brain begins to demand more to produce the same effects.

Because of this, you feel the need to drink more or take more drugs. Your life might start to get out of hand. Nothing more can dominate your thoughts and actions than getting your next fix. Addiction treatment is often necessary to help those who reach this point break their addictions.

HOW DOES THERAPY FOR AMINO ACID ADDICTION WORK?

Abuse of drugs or alcohol depletes your amino acid reserves. When you decide to stop using drugs and alcohol, the withdrawal symptoms you experience are influenced in part by this. Supplements are used in amino acid therapy to replenish your amino acids. Alterations to your diet can also help you feel better and raise your levels of amino acids.

It is not the goal of amino acid therapy to provide a quick fix for addiction. As part of a comprehensive treatment plan that is provided to you during addiction treatment, it works well. To overcome the issues that cause your addiction, you must continue to attend therapy sessions.

A client's genetic test is typically the first step in the treatment. That enables us to estimate the number of modifications in your alleles. Additionally, it reveals whether your genetic predisposition to addiction is genetically determined.

Clients with substance use disorders are offered a full range of treatment options by Coalition Recovery. Our clients stand the best chance of long-term recovery with this strategy.

WHAT ARE THE OPPORTUNITIES FOR AMINO ACID THERAPY?

A mental health condition is often found in the patients who attend Coalition Recovery for addiction treatment. Neurochemical imbalances can be corrected through amino acid therapy, which can also assist in balancing mood disorders' symptoms. When you control your emotions, it can be easier to concentrate on learning techniques that will help you stay sober after addiction treatment.

Mood disorders can be successfully treated with amino acid therapy. It may assist in resolving imbalances in neurochemicals, which in turn may aid in balancing the symptoms of mood disorders. You will be better able to concentrate on learning the strategies that can assist you in remaining sober after leaving addiction treatment if you can control your emotions. Amino acid therapy may ultimately be an essential component of your overall treatment strategy.

Amino acid therapy is customized for each client by Coalition Recovery. Foods and supplements can be added and taken out until we find the right balance. Amino acid therapy's therapeutic benefits can give you more energy and vitality. In addition, having more self-confidence can support you through the remainder of your addiction treatment program.

Discover amino acid therapy at co-op rehabilitation if you have a mood disorder, amino acid therapy might be a good option for you.

Amino acid is a highly recommended therapy for those that may feel helpless especially when they are struggling with drug addiction. Between 40 and 60 percent of people who receive treatment for alcoholism or addiction relapse within a year. You may have a better chance of avoiding relapse if you choose the right addiction therapy.

What is the connection between addiction therapy and amino acids? How might it help you on your way to recovery?

For you to make an educated decision before seeking addiction treatment, we will go over the fundamentals of the connection between amino acids and recovery from addiction in this guide. It's possible that incorporating amino acids into your addiction treatment is precisely what you need.

Learn more by reading on!

How do amino acids work?

Protein makes up about 20% of the human body. Amino acids are the constructive bodies of these proteins.

The fundamental building blocks of all of your cells, hormones, and neurotransmitters are amino acids. Getting enough protein in your diet can help you feel better and perform better in sports.

The human body requires a total of twenty distinct amino acids for growth and function. Nine of these amino acids are essential, necessitating their consumption. The body can synthesize the remaining eleven.

These are the nine essential amino acids:

These amino acids are not made by the body on their own: tryptophan, saline, threonine, methionine, phenylalanine, lysine, Lucien, isoleucine, and histidine are all examples. Instead, you get these amino acids from your diet. Your body breaks down the protein into the specific amino acids found in high-protein foods like poultry, eggs, meat, and legumes. These amino acids can then be used by your body to build important chemicals like neurotransmitters and the structure of your cells.

Amino Acid Therapy: What Is It?

The specialized supplementation of amino acids for addiction recovery is known as amino acid therapy.

Substance abuse frequently results in malnourishment and nutritional imbalances. It's possible that a person who uses drugs or alcohol regularly is not getting enough calories or eating a well-balanced diet. A person taking stimulants, for instance, may go days without eating and have no appetite. Or, a person who drinks a lot may not have enough of the B vitamins that the body needs to break down alcohol.

It is essential to feed the body and make up for any specific nutritional deficiencies during the early stages of recovery. Together, our doctor and nutritionist make sure that we eat a well-balanced diet and take supplements to get the nutrients we need.

Amino acid therapy is made to make sure that people who are struggling with addiction get more of the nutrients they need to recover. The cravings, mood swings, and physical pain of withdrawal from addictive substances can be reduced by providing your body with the necessary amino acids. Amino acids can reduce relapse rates by lessening an addict's dependence on their drug of choice. Amino Acid Therapy for Substance Abuse Recovery at Bridging the Gaps, our primary goal is to heal the person as a whole. Counseling and programs like Alcoholics Anonymous or Narcotics Anonymous address the psychological and spiritual aspects of addiction in traditional treatment. We go one step further by focusing on the physiological aspects of addiction as well.

A brain imbalance of neurotransmitters is the cause of substance dependence. A chemical that moves a signal from one neuron to another is called a neurotransmitter. Multiple neurotransmitter systems may play a significant role in addiction development, according to research.

Remember that neurotransmitters begin with amino acids. We at Bridging the Gaps find and focus on the brain's depleted neurotransmitters that drive substance abuse. The specific nutrients the body needs to make its neurotransmitters and restore brain balance are provided by amino acid therapy.

The Benefits of Amino Acid Therapy Without neurotransmitters and amino acids, neurotransmitter depletion could occur. Among the signs of a lack of neurotransmitters are:

Anxiety Memory loss Sleep disorders Addiction disorders what, then, is the connection between addiction therapy and amino acids?

Serotonin is one type of neurotransmitter. Serotonin's antidepressant properties are well-known, but low levels of this neurotransmitter are linked to alcoholism as well.

Serotonin levels may be low when an individual is recovering from alcohol addiction. Vitamins and the specific amino acids needed for the brain to produce more serotonin are provided by amino acid therapy. The goal of amino acid therapy is to rebuild the mind and body at the cellular level. The brain's normal chemical production might be restored through this process. Reducing cravings can be made easier with stable brain function. Your chances of completing your rehabilitation and recovery could increase if you raise your levels of neurotransmitters.

Why Take a Supplement?

It is not enough to eat and hope your body gets the amino acids it needs in early recovery.

Instead, you can get your body the right amount of amino acids by using amino acid therapy. It's important to talk to a doctor or nurse who can figure out the right nutrients and dosage for your needs.

This process relies heavily on when you take your supplements. Your bloodstream's circulating amino acids become depleted in the time between meals. Between meals, bridging the Gaps provides additional protein to ensure that amino acids are readily available. Your mood and energy levels will be more stable when your body gets the nutrients it needs consistently.

Addiction can be treated with amino acids by treating withdrawal symptoms. You can make sure that your body gets the specific amino acids it needs to reduce the abstinence symptoms that come with quitting drugs and alcohol.

Amino Acids and Treatment for Addiction Prepare yourself for Success. You can give your body the building blocks it needs for a successful recovery with amino acid therapy. Today, learn more about addiction therapy and amino acids!

Are you finding it difficult to make a decision concerning your addiction problem? We are here to assist. We focus on addiction's underlying causes to create a path to wellness or out of control can find hope at our Tampa Bay facility. People in need receive assistance from Coalition Recovery:

There are series of drug and alcohol recovery treatment Intervention programs Detox programs

CHAPTER SEVEN

The Physical Allergy of Addiction and Alcohol The physical allergy of addiction to drugs or alcohol can be difficult to accept oneself. This is because the physical allergy of addiction is what permanently makes us addicts and alcoholics. Our physical allergy is what distinguishes us from others; our physical characteristics are in comparison to recreational or "normal" drinkers. It is used in science to explain how addicts and alcoholics process substances in different ways, how our brains react to them, and how our bodies are made uniquely.

Numerous issues for which we have never had an answer before recent studies can be explained by this. The reason you can't stop yourself from using after just one drink is the physical allergy of addiction. Even though you tell yourself you wouldn't, it's the reason you keep using the same substance. It's the allergy that makes you spend money you promised not to spend regularly and causes you to pass out while drinking instead of sticking to the one or two drinks you promised.

Your cravings are brought on by the allergy that underlies your addiction.

Any Substance Allergy or physical allergy is very similar to any other allergy we may encounter in our lives. What is an allergy?" A damaging immune response by the body to a substance" is an allergy. Milk and dust would be two examples. When lactose-intolerant individuals consume dairy products, they experience an allergic reaction and exhibit abnormal responses; they get very sick. When we consume alcohol or drugs, just like an addict or alcoholic, we experience an abnormal response, and that abnormal response is a desire for more; we must continue. The reason for this is that for "normal" drinkers and drug users, the response is to get out of control, and they get sick, causing them to want to stop or be able to stop. Most people's typical reaction to drugs or alcohol is to stop after a certain point.

Whether we're an alcoholic or drug addicts, we never give up, no matter what happens. What's going on? We are allergic to these substances as a result of our allergy. As addicts, the allergic response we experience is a constant desire for more, which forces us to relinquish control and allow the substance to exert its influence over us. Drugs and alcohol give us the impression of being in charge, forcing us to do anything to get more and keep going so we don't get sick. The allergy begins to take effect as soon as you take your first drink or use a drug.

Oddly, these substances cause different reactions in different people, but no brain is wired the same way. We all have very different inner makeup as a result of our distinct outer makeup.

Without this knowledge and comprehension, many of us go about our daily lives assuming that we are just bad people and that we are not strong enough people to stop doing things that hurt us. We have been able to make so many poor choices in our lives without thinking about the consequences because we believe our bodies are sickened by this allergy. We never intended to harm ourselves or anyone else, but the allergy to this disease made us see past everything; it has complete control over our lives. Take this as the missing piece of the puzzle and put it to work for your sobriety. You are not malicious. You are not in any way weak. You are unique, and that is perfectly acceptable.

An allergic reaction to a medication is known as a drug allergy. The drug causes an allergic reaction in your immune system, which fights infection and disease. Symptoms of this reaction include a rash, a high temperature, and difficulty breathing.

True drug allergies are rare. An actual drug allergy accounts for less than 5% to 10% of adverse drug reactions. The remainder is drug-related side effects. However, knowing if you have a drug allergy and what to do about it is essential.

Subscribe to our weekly Allergies & Asthma email to receive expert advice and treatment news to assist you in avoiding triggers and managing reactions.

Please enter your email address to subscribe to our popular Heart Health newsletter. Your privacy is important to us.

Your immune system helps keep you healthy. It is made to fight foreign invaders like parasites, viruses, bacteria, and other harmful substances. Your immune system misidentifies a drug that enters your body as one of these invaders when you have a drug allergy. Your immune system initiates the production of antibodies in response to what it considers to be a threat. These are particular proteins that have been programmed to fight the invader. They target the drug in this instance.

Inflammation rises as a result of this immune response, which can manifest as a rash, fever, or difficulty breathing. The immune response may occur the very first time you take the medication, or it may not occur until after you have taken it numerous times without experiencing any issues.

Is it always risky to have a drug allergy?

Sometimes not. A drug allergy might not cause you to notice any symptoms at all. You may only get a mild rash.

However, a serious drug allergy can be fatal. It might lead to anaphylaxis. A sudden, life-threatening, all-body reaction to a drug or other allergen is called anaphylaxis. Within minutes of taking the medication, you could experience an anaphylactic reaction. In some instances, it may occur 12 hours after taking the drug. Some of the signs include:

Anaphylaxis can be fatal if not treated immediately. irregular heartbeat difficulty breathing swelling unconsciousness after taking a medication, if any of these symptoms occur, call 911 or go to the nearest emergency room.

Reactions resembling anaphylaxis can occur when taking certain medications for the first time. Anaphylactic reactions can be triggered by the following drugs:

Morphine, aspirin, some chemotherapy drugs, and some X-ray dyes. This kind of reaction usually doesn't involve the immune system and isn't an actual allergy. However, it is just as dangerous and has the same symptoms and treatment as true anaphylaxis.

What drugs are most likely to cause drug allergies?

People react differently to various drugs. However, some drugs are more likely than others to trigger allergic reactions. These are some:

Antibiotics like penicillin and sulfa antibiotics like sulfamethoxazole-trimethoprim aspirin nonsteroidal anti-inflammatory medications like ibuprofen anticonvulsants like carbamazepine and lamotrigine medications used in monoclonal antibody therapy like trastuzumab and ibritumomab Tiuxetan chemotherapy drugs like paclitaxel, docetaxel, and pro

Only a few people are affected by a drug allergy. It always has a negative impact and involves the immune system.

However, any drug user can experience a side effect. Additionally, it rarely involves the immune system. Any action of the drug, whether beneficial or harmful, that is unrelated to the drug's primary function is a side effect.

For instance, the painkiller aspirin frequently has the undesirable side effect of causing stomach upset. However, it also reduces your risk of heart attack and stroke, which is a positive side effect. The painkiller acetaminophen (Tylenol) can damage the liver as well. Additionally, nitroglycerin, which is used to increase blood flow and widen blood vessels, may also enhance mental function as a side effect.

Is drug allergic reaction Positive or negative? Either positive or negative who is it affecting? Who specifically involves the immune system? How is a drug allergy treated, rarely but always?

The severity of a drug allergy determines how to treat it. If you have a severe allergic reaction to a drug, you may need to stay away from it completely. Your doctor will likely attempt to substitute a different medication that you are not allergic to.

Your doctor may still prescribe a medication to you even if you have a mild allergic reaction. However, they might also suggest a different medication to help you manage your reaction. The immune system can be suppressed and symptoms reduced by taking certain medications. These are some:

Antihistamines your body produces histamine when it perceives a substance as being harmful, such as an allergen. Histamine release may cause allergic symptoms like swelling, itchiness, or irritation. An antihistamine may help alleviate these allergic reaction symptoms by preventing the production of histamine. Pills, eye drops, creams, and nasal sprays are all forms of antihistamines.

Corticosteroids a drug allergy can result in serious symptoms like swelling of the airways. These issues can be alleviated with the assistance of corticosteroids. Pills, eye drops, nasal sprays, and creams are all forms of corticosteroids. Additionally, they are available as a liquid for injection or use in a nebulizer as well as powder for use in an inhaler.

Bronchodilators your doctor may recommend a bronchodilator if your drug allergy makes you cough or wheeze. This medication will aid in airway opening and ease breathing. Utilizing an inhaler or nebulizer, bronchodilators can be taken as a liquid or as a powder.

What is a person with a drug allergy's long-term outlook?

Over time, your immune system can change. Your allergy might weaken, disappear, or get worse. As a result, it's critical to always follow your doctor's drug management instructions. Be sure to follow their advice to avoid the drug or similar substances.

Talk to your doctor as soon as you notice any signs of a drug allergy or serious side effects from a medication you are taking.

Take the following steps if you are aware that you are allergic to any medication:

Inform each one of your medical professionals. This includes your dentist as well as any other medical professionals who consider carrying a card or displaying your drug allergy on a bracelet or necklace. This information could be you're only ticked from endangering your life in case of an emergency.

If you have any questions about your allergy, talk to your doctor. Some examples might be:

When I take this medication, what kind of allergic reaction should I look for?

Is there anything else I should stay away from because of my allergy?

Should I keep any medications on hand in case I get a reaction?

CHAPTER 8

Herbal Treatments for Drug Addiction According to the American Society of Addiction Medicine (ASAM), addiction is a chronic disease that can be treated. It is caused by complicated interactions between a person's genetics, brain circuits, environment, and life experiences. Despite the negative effects, addicts abuse substances and frequently engage in compulsive behaviors.

Addiction affects over 23 million adults in the United States over the age of 12. Addicts use drugs like heroin, cocaine, prescription drugs, and alcohol. To deal with stress, some people use drugs. Others become addicted as a result of developments like their teenage years or the influence of those around them.

An addict's recovery from addiction requires intervention. When addicts pose a threat to themselves and others, you must assist them. Numerous emotional, health and social issues can result from addiction. It may be necessary to overcome addiction to prevent these difficulties from occurring. You can use a variety of approaches to assist an addict. It is possible to deal with addictions without using any medications with non-drug treatments.

1. For a long time, herbs and their components and derivatives have been essential in the fight against drug abuse. It has been used as traditional medicine by the Chinese, Indians, and Americans.

An image of a man blending leaves in a blender as an alternative to alcohol addiction treatment, alcohol addiction treatment, drug addiction treatment, drug addiction treatment center, and addiction treatment

Kudzu. For nearly a millennium, the Chinese have used this plant to cut down on alcohol consumption. According to a 2005 Harvard University study, participants who took kudzu drank less beer than those who did not. Puerarin, which is found in kudzu, increases blood flow to the brain, which makes people feel better and makes them drink less.

Pueraria RadixThe isoflavone daidzin in this herb slows down alcohol metabolism. Consequently, its effects are comparable to those of disulfiram. Your alcohol consumption will slow as a result of these effects.

Peyote. This herb was used to treat alcohol use disorder by Native Americans. Mescaline in it prevents you from drinking.

Laurifolia thunbergia addicts can avoid alcohol liver toxicity with this herb.

Withania is drowsy. This herb has been shown to reduce morphine tolerance in animal models.

Salvia miltiorrhiza. This herb has been shown in animal models to reduce alcohol consumption.

These herbs may have harmful side effects despite their benefits. Before using them to reduce their effects, you should talk to your doctor about it.

2. Diet According to natural medicine specialists, hypoglycemia is an essential component of alcohol use disorder. Your organs are damaged

and your nutritional status is altered by alcohol and other drugs. Many alcohol addicts are malnourished as a result.

Addicts in recovery require a well-balanced diet that provides the necessary nutrients to repair organ damage. They also get the energy they need from the food to avoid using drugs.

a picture of a woman holding an apple, healthy foods, healthy places to eat near me, healthy eating near me, and a healthy eating plan Small, well-balanced meals are recommended throughout the day. Fresh fruits, lean animal protein, nuts, whole grains, and vegetables are all essential components of an addict's diet. Alcoholics must regularly consume these foods and pay attention to them. They are in place of the alcoholic beverages they consumed to satiate their stomachs. Additionally, the food will maintain their glucose levels.

Many substance withdrawal symptoms include insomnia. You can get some sleep by having a snack of chicken or turkey. They give you tryptophan, which helps you sleep, and serotonin precursor, which helps you sleep.

If you experience hypoglycemia, do not grab a candy bar immediately. Natural foods that maintain a stable blood sugar level should be your priority instead. Refined sugar-containing food items can temporarily raise blood sugar levels significantly. Caffeinated beverages should be avoided because they can make you want to use the substance you're quitting. When addicts of other drugs use alcohol to stop abusing those drugs, this is known as cross-addiction.

3. Addicts working with professionals to identify and alter the behaviors that lead to substance abuse is a natural treatment known as behavioral counseling. The expert looks at how addicts live their lives and comes up with the right treatment plan to help them deal with or avoid triggers, change how they feel about drugs, and improve their health.

The addict can try one of two behavioral treatment options.

a. Outpatient Behavioral Counseling: In this method, the addict meets with the counselor at their home within the allotted time frame. The patient can see the expert on their own or with a group of people who are going through the same problems. The following types of outpatient behavioral treatment are provided by professionals:

Rewards are used as motivational incentives to encourage drug abstinence. Every achievement the recovering addict makes receives positive reinforcement. They look forward to the next important step to earn the next prize because of this reward.

The duration of motivational interviews is brief. It aims to motivate people to alter their drug abuse patterns. The participants determine the potential advantages and disadvantages of ending addiction. Additionally, they devise strategies for ensuring that the recovering addict adheres to the program.

Family members and the addict are both involved in multidimensional family therapy. It aims to address the issue collectively. This treatment includes addressing the issues brought on by drug abuse. It also tries to find the right framework to help addicts recover.

The therapist works with an individual or small group during cognitive behavioral therapy. It pinpoints the circumstances and emotions that contribute to drug abuse. The treatment aims to modify your response to these triggers.

b. Residential Behavioral Treatment In this method, the addict is admitted to a facility to receive treatment for a predetermined amount of time. Patients with severe substance use disorders find it convenient. While keeping an eye on the patient's progress, the experts can offer advice.

Before being allowed to leave the facilities, patients must complete intensive treatment plans.

How is drug addiction treated with behavioral therapies?

Addiction treatment with behavioral therapy is highly effective. Experts learn from addicts' experiences. The professionals take note of their accounts and devise a strategy to assist them in overcoming their addiction. The following issues are enclosed in the program:

Addicts' attitudes toward drug use shift as a result of the treatment. They emphasize the causes of addiction as well as the consequences for addicts and their loved ones. They may be able to stop using drugs thanks to this revelation.

It makes your health better. The therapists advise patients on what to avoid and how to get fitter.

Treatment plans are accepted. Addicts in recovery are guided in following their recovery plans by experts. They tell them about the obstacles they might have to overcome and the consequences if they don't. They are more open to their recovery when they are aware.

4. Supplements for nutrition Addiction has an impact on how your organs work. Addicts don't take care of themselves, and the drugs they use may contain harmful ingredients that harm their bodies. The liver, kidney, and heart are just a few of the body's organs that are affected by drugs.

Your health depends on these particular parts of your body. Changing how they work can have serious consequences, like illnesses that can kill you.

Addicts Should Take the Following Supplements While Recovering, Say Experts:

Your digestive system gets a boost from the vitamin B complex. This improvement assists your body in metabolizing and absorbing food nutrients. Anxiety and insomnia can be alleviated with pyridoxine (B6). The B1 vitamin thiamine aids in thinking and recalling.

Minerals aid in the treatment of a mineral deficiency caused by addiction. Calcium and magnesium improve bone health, nerve function, and the muscle system, as well as reduce irritability. Zinc is essential for addicts' liver, brain, and immune systems. Addicts benefit from iron, potassium, and selenium.

Because of your addiction and poor diet, Omega-3 provides essential nutrients that may be lacking in your body.Omega-3 may also help with irritability, inflammation, depression, and anxiety.

The nutrients you consume are transported and stored by amino acids. Various substance addicts have benefited greatly from specific amino acids. D-phenylalanine treats heroin, alcohol, marijuana, and tobacco addicts, while L-glutamine helps alcohol addicts.

5. Acupuncture a treatment method that has been around for a long time is acupuncture. To combat cravings and withdrawal symptoms, the Chinese inserted needles into their skin. The piercing brings the body back into balance. Acupuncture has been proven to assist addicts conquer drug addiction and withdrawal symptoms like pain.

To fully comprehend acupuncture, additional research is required. Addicts are encouraged to try acupuncture under the supervision of a licensed professional. It would be helpful if you didn't try it on your own.

6. Yoga has numerous advantages Sessions teach patients about drug abuse, give them advice, and show them how to deal with the urge to use drugs. For people with mild addictions, outpatient behavioral counseling is a good option. It doesn't disrupt your routine and is frequently less expensive. However, compared to residential treatment, it has a lower success rate.

Remembering that addiction is a disease that can be treated is important for addicts. They are not weak because they are dependent on drugs. Drug addiction affects approximately 23 million Americans; you won't be alone. Utilizing these strategies, you can overcome your substance abuse disorder. Recovery is difficult, but with the right mindset, approach, and support, you can overcome substance abuse.

CONCLUSION

 Many Americans are affected by drug addiction. Sadly, the threat has repercussions for addicts and those around them. The good news is that you can kick your drug addiction. Although the process is time-consuming, these non-drug treatments work.

Your recovery depends on your diet and behavioral therapy. Your view of drugs changes as a result of behavioral therapy. You will have the strength and nutrients you need to resist the urge to use drugs if you eat a well-balanced diet. Yoga and acupuncture are great alternatives for overcoming addiction.

The professionals at Ascendant New York Drug and Alcohol Detox can assist you. During your stay at the detox center, you will receive support through residential treatment. You can take advantage of their round-the-clock care with this strategy.

As you continue with your life, you will receive occasional assistance from Ascendant New York

Drug and Alcohol Detox as part of outpatient treatment. With Ascendant's rehab in New York, there is always hope that drug abuse can be cured.